THE ULTIMATE WORKOUT PLAN FOR BUSY WOMEN

Transform Your Body in Just 30 Days

Dr. Rachel Ferguson

TABLE OF CONTENTS

Contact Us:

You can also contact us in our 24hrs email address for guidance or advice.
mailto:drrachelferguson@gmail.com

Reach out below to see more of our health books and lots more in our store!

Drrachelferguson

Appreciation

We would be forever grateful if you could take a few moments after you've finished reading, to leave us a positive review on Amazon. Your review will not only help us to reach a wider audience, but it will also help other readers to discover the value of our book. We know that your time is valuable, so we truly appreciate your willingness to share your thoughts with us. Thank you in advance for your kind review.

INTRODUCTION

Mental preparation and motivation

Set your mindset for success by visualizing your goals and the benefits of completing the 30-day workout plan.

Establish a support system by sharing your fitness journey with family or friends who can provide encouragement and accountability.

Create a motivational playlist or find podcasts that inspire and energize you during workouts.

Prioritize self-care activities such as quality sleep, stress management, and proper nutrition to support your fitness endeavors.

Setting realistic goals and expectations

Assess your starting point: Take an honest look at your current fitness level, strengths, and areas for improvement.

Consider factors such as endurance, strength, flexibility, and body composition.

Define specific goals: Set clear and measurable goals that are specific to your needs and desires. For example, aim to increase strength by lifting a certain weight, improve cardiovascular endurance by running a certain distance, or lose a specific amount of weight.

Make goals attainable: Ensure your goals are realistic and achievable within the 30-day timeframe. Consider your lifestyle, time availability, and other commitments. Setting overly ambitious goals can lead to frustration and burnout.

Break goals into smaller milestones: Divide your larger goal into smaller, manageable milestones to track your progress and stay motivated.

For example, if your goal is to lose 10 pounds in 30 days, set smaller targets of 2-3 pounds per week.

Set SMART goals: Make your goals Specific, Measurable, Attainable, Relevant, and Time-bound. This framework helps you clarify and refine your goals to increase the likelihood of success.

Consider non-scale victories: Remember that fitness achievements extend beyond the numbers on a scale. Consider other markers of progress, such as increased energy levels, improved sleep, enhanced mood, or fitting into smaller clothing sizes.

Embrace flexibility: Recognize that progress may not always be linear, and setbacks or challenges can occur. Be adaptable and adjust your goals or approach if necessary, without losing sight of the bigger picture.

Be patient and realistic: Understand that significant transformations take time and consistency. Avoid comparing your progress to others and focus on your own journey. Celebrate each milestone achieved along the way.

.

Establishing a Routine Week 1

Day 1: Strength exercises for the whole body

- Start by doing 5–10 minutes of easy cardio.
- Perform complex movements, such as squats, lunges, push-ups, rows, and overhead presses that target the large muscular groups.
- Perform 2-3 sets of 8–12 repetitions for each exercise, using good form and slow, deliberate motions.
- Rest for 30 to 60 seconds in between sets.
- To increase flexibility, stretch for 5 to 10 minutes to wind down.

Exercise your heart on day two

- Pick a cardiovascular exercise you like to do, such running, cycling, or utilizing an elliptical machine.
- Begin with a 5 minute, moderately paced warm-up.
- Intensify for 20 to 30 minutes, aiming for a demanding but manageable degree of exertion.
- As a cool-down, gradually reduce the intensity during the last five minutes.
- Stretch the main muscle groups to ease tension after exercise and speed up recovery.

Day 3: A day of active rest

- Take part in low-impact exercises like Pilates, yoga, or gentle stretching.
- Concentrate on enhancing your balance, flexibility, and awareness.
- Keep up your activity level while allowing your body to rest and regenerate.
- To reduce stress, think about adding deep breathing techniques or meditation.

Exercise for the upper body on day four

- Warm up with dynamic upper body stretches or mild aerobics.
- Use movements like the bench press, bent-over rows, shoulder presses, and bicep curls to target the upper body muscles, such as the chest, back, shoulders, and arms.
- Carry out two to three sets of eight to twelve repetitions for each exercise, progressively increasing the weight as needed.
- Rest for 30 to 60 seconds in between sets.
- Finish with stretches that concentrate on the muscles of the upper body.

Physical activity on day five

- Pick a new cardio exercise from Day 2 to mix things up and work various muscle groups.
- Use the same structure as Day 2, including warm-up, sustained exertion, and cool-down intervals.
- Set a goal for yourself to maintain or boost your prior cardio session's intensity or length.

Day 6: A day of active rest

- Select a low-impact exercise that encourages rest and healing, such as restorative yoga, swimming, or gentle strolling.
- Pay attention to muscular discomfort reduction and active healing.
- Use self-massage or foam rolling methods to relieve tension and boost circulation.

Day 7: Strength exercises for the lower body

- Warm up with mild aerobic or active lower body stretches.
- Use movements like squats, lunges, deadlifts, and calf raises to target the lower body's muscles, such as the quadriceps, hamstrings, glutes, and calves.

- Carry out two to three sets of eight to twelve repetitions for each exercise, progressively boosting weight or resistance as needed.
- Rest for 30 to 60 seconds in between sets.
- Lower body stretches should be performed after exercise to increase flexibility and avoid muscular stiffness.
- Set up a dependable regimen that include both strength training and aerobic activity throughout the first week. To aid in recuperation and avoid overtraining, permit active rest days. To lower the danger, make sure to properly warm up and cool down.

Increasing Intensity in Week 2

Day 8: Forty minutes of full-body strength exercise with heavier weights

- 5 minutes of dynamic stretching and gentle cardio serve as the warm-up.
- Use heavier weights than in Week 1 while doing complex exercises including squats deadlifts, bench presses, shoulder presses, and rows.
- With good form and control, aim for three sets of 8–10 repetitions for each exercise.
- Lunges, push-ups, and lat pulldowns are a few examples of exercises that work the primary muscular groups.
- 5 minutes of static stretching for the cool-down.

Day 9: 25-minute HIIT exercise with longer intervals

- 5 minutes of brisk aerobic and dynamic stretches serve as the warm-up.
- Exercises that need a high level of intensity include burpees, mountain climbers, jumping jacks, and squat jumps.

- 45 seconds of vigorous activity and 15 seconds of rest should be alternated.
- Plan on 4-5 rounds of short, sharp intervals.
- 5 minutes of easy cardio and static stretching make up the cool-down.

Yoga or Pilates on Day 10

- Attend a yoga or Pilates class to strengthen your core and improve your flexibility.
- Stretching sore muscles, increasing the mind-body connection, and correcting posture should all be priorities.
- Investigate different yoga forms, such as Vinyasa, Hatha, or Yin.
- Use relaxation methods and deep breathing.
- Pick a session based on your interests and skill level.

Day 11: 35 minutes of more intense cardiovascular activity

- Pick a cardio exercise you like, like jogging, cycling, or utilizing an elliptical machine.
- By increasing the inclination, resistance, or speed, the intensity may be raised.
- Throughout the workout, strive to maintain an effort of a moderate to high intensity.

- By alternating between intensities that are greater and lower, include interval training.
- 5 minutes of easy cardio and static stretching make up the cool-down.

Day 12: 30 minutes of upper body-focused strength training

- 5 minutes of dynamic stretching and easy cardio constitute the warm-up.
- Concentrate on upper body workouts including push-ups, dumbbell curls, tricep dips, and shoulder lifts.
- Use weights that are difficult for you and aim for three sets of 8–10 repetitions for each exercise.
- To increase effectiveness, use circuit training or supersets.
- 5 minutes of static stretching for the cool-down.

Day 13: 25-minute HIIT workout with a variety of exercises

- 5 minutes of brisk aerobic and dynamic stretches serve as the warm-up.
- Mix high-intensity workouts that target several muscle groups into your workout.

- Include exercises like lateral lunges, plank variants, kettle bell swings, and squat thrusts.
- 40 seconds of vigorous activity and 20 seconds of rest should be alternated.
- Plan on 4-5 rounds of short, sharp intervals.
- 5 minutes of easy cardio and static stretching make up the cool-down.

Day 14: Day of rest

- Give your body time to heal and regenerate.
- Put your attention on self-care practices like calming baths, foam rolling, and gentle stretching.
- Attend to any muscular discomfort or exhaustion by paying attention to your body.
- Take advantage of today to evaluate your development and get ready for the following week.

Week 3: Focusing on Particular Areas

Day 15: 45 minutes of circuit-style strength training for the entire body

- 5 minutes of dynamic stretching and easy cardio constitute the warm-up.
- Exercises targeting various muscle groups, such as squats, lunges, push-ups, rows, and planks, should be done in a circuit.
- For each exercise, aim for 3 sets of 10–12 reps with little to no rest in between.
- Pick weights that will push you while still enabling proper form and control.
- Include activities that strengthen the core and advance stability all around.
- 5 minutes of static stretching for the cool-down.

Bodyweight exercises and cardiovascular exercise for 40 minutes on Day 16

- 5 minutes of brisk aerobic and dynamic stretches serve as the warm-up.
- Alternate between bodyweight exercises and cardio exercises (such as jogging, cycling, or using a cardio machine).
- Exercises like jumping jacks, burpees, mountain climbers, and bodyweight squats should be done.
- For each bodyweight exercise, aim for 3–4 sets of 12–15 repetitions.
- Depending on your level of fitness, change the length and intensity of your cardio intervals.
- 5 minutes of easy cardio and static stretching make up the cool-down.

Day 17: An active rest day (light yoga or stretching).

- Engage in a stretching or mild yoga practice to increase flexibility, mobility, and relaxation.
- Focus on stretching main muscle groups and regions of tension.

- Include yoga postures that target particular sections of the body, such as forward folds, lunges, twists, and hip openers.
- Practice deep breathing and mindfulness to decrease stress and increase mental well-being.
- Choose a session that helps you to relax and replenish your body.

Day 18: HIIT workout with advanced exercises (30 minutes)

- 5 minutes of brisk aerobic and dynamic stretches serve as the warm-up.
- Incorporate tough and advanced routines into your HIIT regimen.
- Include workouts like burpee variants, plyometric leaps, kettle bell swings, and sprints.
- 30 seconds of all-out exertion followed by 15 seconds of recovery should be alternated.
- Focus on 5–6 rounds of short, sharp intervals.
- 5 minutes of easy cardio and static stretching make up the cool-down.

Day 19: Strength exercise focused on core muscles (35 minutes)

- 5 minutes of dynamic stretching and easy cardio constitute the warm-up.
- Perform workouts that target the core, such as planks, Russian twists, bicycle crunches, and stability ball exercises.
- Aim for 3 sets of 10-12 repetitions for each exercise, concentrating on perfect form and utilizing the core muscles.
- Include activities that test stability and balance, such as single-leg exercises or stability ball exercises.
- 5 minutes of static stretching for the cool-down.

Day 20: Cardiovascular exercise with varied equipment (40 minutes)

- 5 minutes of brisk aerobic and dynamic stretches serve as the warm-up.
- Pick a different piece of cardio equipment or cardiovascular exercise than you usually do (such as a rowing machine, stair climber, or swimming).

- Decide on a difficult intensity or resistance level and strive to maintain that effort for the whole session.
- To keep the exercise interesting, include interval training or different intensities.
- 5 minutes of easy cardio and static stretching make up the cool-down.

Day 21: Day of rest

- Give your body a day off from strenuous exercise to heal and repair.
- Use today to unwind, practice self-care, or engage in active healing activities like brisk walking or mild stretching.
- Reflect

Week 4: Pushing the Boundaries

Day 22: Strength training for the whole body with more repetitions and sets (50 minutes)

- 5 minutes of dynamic stretching and easy cardio constitute the warm-up.
- By increasing the number of repetitions and sets in your strength training routines, you may up the intensity.
- For each exercise, aim for 4 sets of 10–12 repetitions while pushing yourself with heavier weights or more difficult variants.
- To work many muscle groups, mix complex workouts with isolation ones.
- During each repeat, keep your form correct and concentrate on connecting your muscles and thoughts.
- 5 minutes of static stretching for the cool-down.

Day 23: A 35-minute advanced HIIT workout that includes plyometrics

- 5 minutes of brisk aerobic and dynamic stretches serve as the warm-up.
- Include plyometric and explosive movements in your HIIT regimen.
- Perform exercises including lateral bounds, box jumps, tuck jumps, and burpee variants.
- 40 seconds of all-out exertion and 20 seconds of recovery should be alternated.
- Intensify your intervals by pushing yourself to leap higher and move quicker for 5–6 rounds.
- 5 minutes of easy cardio and static stretching make up the cool-down.

Day 24: A restful day of activity (yoga or Pilates)

- Attend a yoga or Pilates class to improve your flexibility, balance, and awareness of your body.

- To increase general strength and mobility, concentrate on deep stretches, balancing postures, and controlled movements.
- If you feel comfortable and it is appropriate for your level of competence, include hard yoga positions like inversions or arm balances.
- To decrease stress and enhance mental health, try mindfulness and relaxation practices.
- Select a workout that enables you to recover and become ready for the next sessions.

Cardiovascular activity for 45 minutes that is longer in length and more intense.

- 5 minutes of brisk aerobic and dynamic stretches serve as the warm-up.
- Increase the length of your cardio workout while keeping the intensity at a greater level.
- Spend a lot of time exercising, such as jogging, cycling, or swimming.

- By include intervals, hills, or sprints in the program, the intensity may be raised.
- Aim for a prolonged effort that tests your ability to withstand physical stress.
- 5 minutes of easy cardio and static stretching make up the cool-down.

Day 26: Forty minutes of strength training with an emphasis on functional movements

- 5 minutes of dynamic stretching and easy cardio constitute the warm-up.
- Place a focus on movements-like exercises that increase functional strength.
- Include exercises like push-ups, squats, lunges, deadlifts, and swings with a kettle bell.
- Exercises for stability and balance should be included, such as single-leg poses or medicine ball exercises.

- Aim for three sets of 10–12 repetitions, performed carefully and with good technique.
- 5 minutes of static stretching for the cool-down.

Day 27: 35-minute, difficult HIIT exercise with extra resistance

- 5 minutes of brisk aerobic and dynamic stretches serve as the warm-up.
- Introduce resistance tools into your HIIT exercise, such as resistance bands, dumbbells, or kettle bells.
- Perform exercises like resistance band lateral walks, squat presses, bicep curls, and renegade rows.
- 30 seconds of all-out exertion followed by 15 seconds of recovery should be alternated.
- Push yourself to increase resistance and pace as you attempt 5–6 rounds of hard interval training.
- 5 minutes of easy cardio and static stretching make up the cool-down.

Day 28: Day of rest

- Give your body time to rest and refuel in preparation for the difficulties ahead.
- Take part in

Week 5: Upholding and Considering

Day 29: 45 minutes of full-body strength exercise at the same pace as the previous day

- 5 minutes of dynamic stretching and easy cardio constitute the warm-up.

- Your full-body strength training regimen should be continued with the same weights and intensity as in Week 4.
- For each exercise, aim for 3–4 sets of 10–12 repetitions, paying close attention to maintaining perfect form and control.
- Squeezing the targeted muscles while concentrating on the mind-muscle connection will challenge you.
- To guarantee a tough exercise while keeping proper technique, adjust weights as necessary.
- 5 minutes of static stretching for the cool-down.

Cardiovascular activity for 40 minutes on day 30 at the same intensity.

- 5 minutes of brisk aerobic and dynamic stretches serve as the warm-up.
- Maintain a consistent effort while continuing with the same aerobic exercise and intensity as in Week 4.

- Maintain appropriate form, pay attention to your breathing, and exert yourself to the required degree of intensity.

- If you feel comfortable doing so, attempt to gently increase the time or intensity to keep yourself challenged.

- 5 minutes of easy cardio and static stretching make up the cool-down.

Honor accomplishments and consider progress

Take time during the 30-day training schedule to reflect on and congratulate your successes.

Think back on your progress, your accomplishments, and the difficulties you overcame.

To keep track of your accomplishments, think about taking measurements, taking pictures, or keeping a diary.

Recognize the advantages exercise has for both your physical and emotional health.

Motivate yourself to continue pursuing your health and fitness goals by using this reflection.

Create new objectives to continue your fitness journey

Setting new objectives comes after reflecting on your progress and celebrating your accomplishments.

Decide on the areas you wish to develop, whether it be your strength, endurance, flexibility, or willingness to try new things.

Achieve your dreams by setting SMART (specific, measurable, achievable, relevant, and time-bound) goals.

To make your objectives more attainable and measurable, break them down into smaller milestones.

To assist you in creating a unique strategy for continuous improvement, take into consideration asking a fitness expert or trainer for advice.

Conclusion

In conclusion, this 30-day workout plan for busy women is designed to provide a powerful and effective framework for incorporating exercise into a busy lifestyle. By progressively increasing intensity, targeting specific areas, pushing limits, and maintaining consistency, you can achieve significant improvements in strength, cardiovascular endurance, and overall fitness.

Throughout the plan, it is essential to prioritize proper warm-up and cool-down routines to prevent injury and optimize performance. Remember to listen to your body, adjust exercises and weights as needed, and focus on maintaining good form and control. Additionally, pay attention to nutrition, hydration, and sufficient rest to support your body's recovery and fuel your workouts.

As you progress through the plan, take time to reflect on your achievements and celebrate the progress you've made. Use this reflection as motivation to set new goals and continue your fitness journey beyond the initial 30 days. Seek guidance from fitness professionals or trainers if needed and remember that fitness is a lifelong commitment.

Stay dedicated, remain consistent, and enjoy the process of becoming a healthier, stronger, and more confident version of yourself. You have the power to achieve your fitness goals, and this workout plan is just the beginning of your transformative journey. Keep pushing forward and embrace the positive changes that come with an active and balanced lifestyle.